Dash Diet Easy Recipes

Easy Recipes for Healthy and Tasty Meal to Improve your Energy and your Wellness

Tom Connor

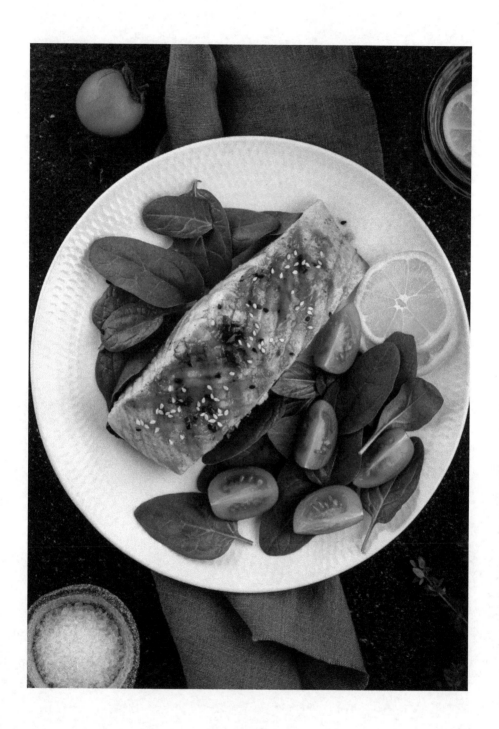

Contents

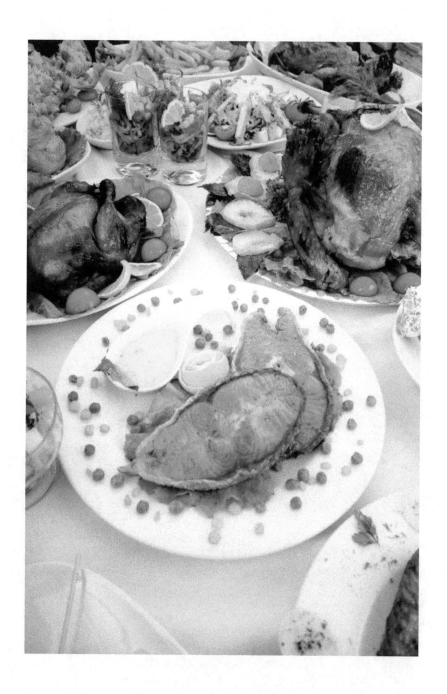

Introduction

The Dash Diet has proven to be one of the healthiest, most effective diets out there that have benefits in a lot of different health-related areas. From cancer to type 2 diabetes, from coronary heart disease to overall immunity enhancement and many more, diet-related problems. Dash diet has the power to prevent and even reverse some of the just mentioned diseases.

The Dash Diet has proven to be one of the healthiest, most effective diets out there that works not only to lower the body's blood pressure but to ensure weight loss, as well. When taking the first steps on a new diet program, however, it can be overwhelming to try and come up with meal ideas and recipes that will keep you in shape and in line with the diet. However, this does not have to be as daunting an experience as you think, which is why this e-book featuring "Dash Diet & 21 Days Dash Diet Meal Plan" is perfect for you. You now have a comprehensive list of delicious, healthy, Dash Diet-friendly meals you can prepare every day for an entire year! This book will allow you to discover all of the benefits of Dash Diet cooking and will even help you to discover some new meals that will quickly become your favorites.

DASH is an acronym for Dietary Approaches to Stop Hypertension, which was the name of the original study. The study organizers wanted to take the best elements of vegetarian diets, which were known to be associated with lower blood pressure, and design a plan that would be flexible enough to appeal to the vast majority of Americans, who are dedicated meat eaters. They developed what they believed was the healthiest omnivore diet plan. And the research has borne out this hope. The DASH diet helps lower blood pressure as well as the first-line medication for hypertension. It also lowers cholesterol. When evaluated over very long periods of time, the DASH eating pattern has been shown to help lower the risk for many diseases and life-threatening medical conditions or events, including stroke, heart attack, heart failure, type 2 diabetes, kidney disease, kidney stones, and some types of cancer. Not only is DASH recommended for people who have these conditions or are at risk for them, but it is recommended for everyone in the Dietary Guidelines for Americans. And the DASH diet is fabulous for weight loss, since it is loaded with bulky, filling fruits and vegetables and has plenty of protein to provide satiety.

Unfortunately, most people who are reading this book haven't noticed any major health problems as of yet, and their main concern is their current shape and how to make it better in a specific period of time. Fortunately for you, you will lose weight fast and naturally while following the Dash diet approach we represent in this book.

While still speaking about a perfect shape, it is also worth mentioning you will also be able to build lean mass and achieve any other fitness-oriented goal you want.

Along with meal plan, you will discover a huge variety of over 100 delicious Dash Diet recipes that will make you excited every time you cook or make your meal prep for the next days. Breakfast, lunch, dinner, various healthy snacks, and side-dishes will definitely satisfy your taste. And even if you have no previous cooking experience, this book also has recipes with less than 5 ingredients to start.

So don't wait, start your new healthy lifestyle right now!

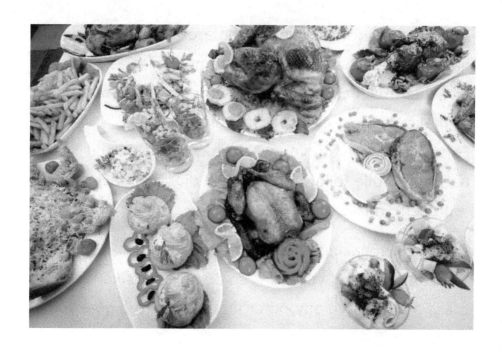

CHAPTER 1

The Psychology of Diet Preparation

Since we have numerous reasons, we resolve to lose weight: we don't like how we look, our clothes don't match, our wellbeing is in danger, the others are wandering, and our work is in danger, or our children are humiliated. We generally think about weight loss as something that only includes our body; definitely, no one has ever wanted to lose weight due to a fat brain or a bloated intellect.

But "we decide" is a function of the mind. It depends on our minds and not on our bodies when and why we take such a decision. We will decide whether we are five pounds heavier than we want, or after two hundred pounds and real medical obesity has passed. The actual body size does not cause the option of losing weight, as this is achieved in the brain.

Since the start (and follow-up) of a dietary program is a mental operation, it seems worth exploring what factors such decisions might cause.

1. Self-Image.

- one of us has a dual picture: our face to the world and our inner idea of how we look. Although we dress and groom to be seen by others as desirable, we are far less affected by others than by our satisfaction or disappointment with us.

Explore this idea by looking at yourself and others over the next week. You will find you are always complimented on the clothes you wear that you don't feel right. Wear a favorite costume perfectly suited, that you think looks amazing and that makes you particularly feel stirring - and nobody notices! The same thing happens with a hairstyle. One morning, you can't get your hair to do something, hurried for time, so you can pull it back with clips with frustration, and hope no one important is looking so bad. That's it! Three people say they like what you did with your hair.

When it comes to our weight, there is the same disconnect. When we look good in our eyes, we don't feel overweight, even though friends and colleagues gossip about our steady increase in weight. However, if we feel overweight, no reassurance from those around us will make us feel less fat. This mental image of our body size, taken to the extreme, can lead to anorexia Nervosa in eating disorders where excessively thin individuals keep their caloric intake dangerously reduced because they constantly feel too large.

We then decide to take a diet in response to our internal self-image. Some of the advantages that we expect are lean and fit take into account others: I'll be more attractive to the opposite

14

sex; I will be noted when it comes to promotion at work; my family and friends will be jealous and have to reassess me as a stronger person than they thought. But what it does for us individually is the true incentive for getting in shape. It is the need to feel better about ourselves, which leads us to diet and exercise through pain and Monotony. It is the vision of us in the future that leads us to our target. Losing this hope or concluding, we won't feel that much better about ourselves are the reasons we give up and slip into the relative convenience of "okay." settling.

2. Body versus Mind dominance.

We all fight for a lifelong inner struggle between our mind and body. Each stage of development is dominant. As kids, we are just a series of sensations. We discover the exciting new world around us by touching everything within reach, sampling everything we can put in our mouths, looking around at the gestures and all the sounds we hear, until finally, we learn to mimic them.

When we step into our early years of education, we begin to reflect on our minds. We eat vast quantities of knowledge voraciously. We learn to read, and our planet extends its borders by 1000 percent. We learn to use the internet, and we have an infinite world at hand.

Then we pass into puberty, and our beauty becomes the primary factor of daily life overnight. We sail through the pitfalls and joys of adolescence, where success and coolness are much more important than learning or mental growth. We spend a very long time on our bodies. We're trying new clothing, new hairstyles, and new maquillage. We have pierced body parts and are exposed to tattoo discomfort because it would make us stand out. We primp, groom, and push ourselves into the models that have been judged by our peers as in."

When we mature, we aspire to reconcile our physical and mental selves. While our corps is supreme in the world of attracting one, we need to practice our minds to advance our careers and establish deep relationships that go far beyond physical attraction.

When we settle down and start creating the good life we want, our energies and efforts turn to things outside of us: children, significant others, friends, family, and jobs. We have so much going on around us that we lose contact with our bodies and minds. We fall into our own comfort zone where food meets so much of our needs. It eases our tension, alleviates our daily tensions, and makes constant blues endurable. It eats away our social connections. It becomes a crucial part of how we express love for those we love. We always see ourselves as we once were and ignore the love handles and pockets of fat that we strongly overlook parts of our body. Our bodies and our inner image of our bodies are becoming increasingly discordant.

3. Our sense of self-efficacy.

Self-efficacy is a psychological concept to describe the perception of a person that any action they take influences the outcome. It is neither self-confidence nor the assumption that you are capable of doing something, although it can include both. It represents our inner hope that what we do will bring about our desired results.

If we begin a diet, want to shape, or begin to take better care of ourselves is essentially a personal choice that may or may not is made as we have expected. The difference lies in the assumption of success, and it's always easier to go on a path that we expect to be successful than to travel to a target where disappointment is the most likely result.

How do we incorporate these principles to make us lean, healthy, and attractive?

We start by looking at our self-image and how we appear to others. Only telling someone Do you think I'm getting too heavy?" does not work unless you have a brutally frank friend or ask somebody who you don't like. Most of us are culturally trained to save the feelings of others so that the answers to such a question are more respectful than real.

Specific focusing can provide better feedback. Tell others that you have a survey for a class you take. Offer a short one-page questionnaire that allows any friend or colleague to list three adjectives that identify various aspects of your physical appearance. Complete yourself one of the sheets. Make sure the responses are confidential by demanding that no names be used and that someone else gathers the sheets completed.

Once the answers are available, compare them to your own answers and see where the descriptions are different. You might find yourself a little defensive. It's not an exercise to make you feel bad about yourself or to gloat about the unexpected compliments. It is an orchestrated endeavor to help you assess the distance between your self-image and your image in the world. Those areas of divergence are a starting point to overlap the two photos.

After defining areas of work, it is time to draw on the unmistakable power of our wonderful mind to start imposing the structure and organization, which we will have to introduce the desired changes. Our mind can only take us where we want to go if it is supported by confidence in our ability to achieve success. Now is the time to reject any failure expectations. Many failed diet and exercise attempts have been made in the past. Leave the past. Leave the past. We are not destined to continue unproductive behavior. We have the gem of a creation, the human mind, able to do almost everything. If we concentrate on any mission, it will succeed if our concerns and doubts do not interfere.

By exploring our memories, we draw on our optimistic aspirations to build up a long list of past achievements. There can be big benchmarks such as endorsing a campaign we liked, planning a great event, or establishing an intense relationship with ourselves. The smallest personal victories are, however, the most important but are generally easily overlooked or dismissed.

Studies and a strong degree in a challenging class show clearly the ability to produce the results you want. Go for quantity: the day you grinned over someone in a smoky room and finished with a short but beautiful affair; the timing study that no-one expected; the night you spin on ice skates. Continue: make the drill squad, shoot a stolen basket, make your own promotional outfit, dying in a wonderful color in your own bathroom, catch a ball, find new apps on your machine and burn your first CD. The list can be infinite and will linger while you recall snippets of the past that you have been burying for a long time.

Hold this list close and read it on a regular basis. It's your self-effective pep band.

You now know the fields in which you can operate and trust the success of your efforts. You must now identify the internal benefits that good weight loss brings. Feel strong, enjoy step-by-step, and quickly zipping your clothes are quick starters. Unconsciously heading to the pool in a short suit is a fantasy enhancing. Making a sales success with the belief that you look best is a picture you will appreciate as you fall asleep. Having someone you like admires or seeing your rivals, jealously emphasizes your determination and maintains the inconvenience of dieting and the demands of repetitive workout routines.

You know where you are going, you know what it will take, and you know that you will succeed. Your mind is set, just waiting for your decision day. Whenever you choose, you will make a choice because you are now under power.

What is Dash Diet Eating Plan?

The dietary eating plan DASH (Dietary Methods to Stop Hypertension) is one of the non-pharmacological therapies for controlling blood pressure. This involves dietary improvements, which include: low consumption of saturated fat, increased fruit and vegetable intakes, more replaced carbohydrate-containing foods, such as whole-grain products, increased seafood, poultry, and nuts intake. The study has shown that the nutritional plan for DASH has the highest effect on blood pressure and cholesterol reduction compared to normal diets. The result is evident within two weeks!

Downward Calory Tips Intake With DASH Eating Schedule!

1. Increase fruit

An apple holds the doctor away for one day! In the food plan for high blood pressure patients, apple and dried apricots are the best options.

2.Growth of vegetables

Burger! Yes, your blood pressure may increase, even if it's a favorite food for most people. I know it's really difficult for you to avoid eating it. However, I recommend that you weigh 3 ounces of meat rather than 6 ounces in the larger size.

The same goes for limiting chicken consumption by just 2 ounces and with a plate of raw vegetables.

3.Enhance fat-free or fat-free dairy products

For example, common ice cream can be replaced with low-fat yogurt.

Reducing Salts and Sodium

By ingesting more fruit and vegetables in the DASH food plan, the lower amount of sodium has made it possible to consume less salt and sodium. Furthermore, fruit and vegetables are rich in potassium and play a part in lowering high blood pressure. Milk products and fish are other important dietary sources.

Tips for Salt and Sodium Reduction

Restrict food high in salt. It is safer to eat no or low-salt foods.

Increased vegetable consumption.

No salted rice, pasta, or other mixed foods

Remove extra salt from preserved foods, such as tuna or beans preserved in a can.

Dash Diet Eating Plan

What is the food for DASH? The DASH diet literally means nutritional methods to avoid high blood pressure. In the early stages of high blood pressure, people are frequently put on this diet to help regulate blood pressure.

The plan is focused on 2,000 calories a day but can be changed to suit your nutritional needs. The American Heart Association recommends this diet highly because it helps to achieve excellent health in many other ways than hypertension. The most significant ingredients to naturally support hypertension are foods high in potassium, foods with calcium and magnesium.

First of all, the DASH strategy assigns great importance to crops. It is good to add whole wheat pieces of bread, wheat pastes, and whole-grain cereals with 7-8 portions per day as a daily allowance on this schedule. Your whole grain has far more nutritional qualities than those that have more refined sugars.

The DASH diet plan also encourages fruit and vegetables. You must eat four to five portions of this category every day. As you review the DASH diet guide, the author tells you several ways to include your regular servings of fruits and vegetables.

Next to this plan are non-fat and low-fat dairy products. You will have to select skim milk, or at most 1 percent, low fat or unfat cheeses and yogurts.

You have lean meat options after milk. There are small portion sizes, indicating no more than two parts. Healthy options include low-fat frankfurters, skinless chicken, and other meat.

When you come to the section where nuts and seeds are listed, they are permitted but are restricted to only five small portions a week. This included legumes as well.

The plan book on the DASH diet is complete. Since you need the plan to fit your everyday calories, it will show you how. This book will also teach you about healthy ways to eat. Eating out is a real challenge in a diet, but the DASH diet book shows you how.

The strategy contains a portion of the book on workouts and alcoholic drinks as well as ways to help you get out of smoking habits.

Additional medical issues with insulin resistance, cholesterol, and inflammation tend to be beneficial. If you have some of these other medical conditions than hypertension, you should like this meal plan very much.

What You Need To Know About The DASH Diet
Our foods will affect our overall health. A diet rich in unhealthy components such as saturated fats and cholesterol is a healthy way to achieve high blood pressure and other diseases. On the other hand, the right food option will reduce the risk of contracting these diseases.

There is a specific eating plan which has demonstrated lower blood pressure or hypertension. This diet is known as DASH or Nutritional Stop Hypertension Approaches.

The DASH diet was a product of clinical trials performed by scientists from the NHLBI. Researchers have found that a diet that is high in potassium, magnesium, calcium, protein, and fibre and low in fat and cholesterol can reduce high blood pressure significantly.

The study showed that even a diet rich in fruits, vegetables, and low-fat milk products has a major influence on hypertension reduction. It also showed that the DASH diet results easily, often in just two weeks from the beginning of the diet.

Three essential nutrients are also stressed by the DASH diet: magnesium, calcium, and potassium. These minerals are intended to minimize hypertension. A standard 2000-calorie diet includes 500 mg of magnesium, 4,7 g of potassium, and 1,2 g of calcium.

Doing the DASH Diet

It is very easy to follow the DASH diet and takes a little time to pick and prepare meals. Foods high in cholesterol and fats are stopped. Dieters should eat as much as possible of vegetables, fruits, and cereals.

Because the foods you consume in a DASH diet are high in fiber content, you can slowly increase your fiber-rich food intake to help prevent diarrhea and other digestive problems. By consuming an additional portion of fruit and vegetables with every meal, you will steadily increase your fiber intake.

Grains are also healthy sources of fiber and vitamins, and minerals of the B-complex. Whole grains, whole wheat bread, bran, wheat germs, and low-fat cereal are all grain items that you can consume to improve your intake of fiber.

You can select the food you consume by looking at processed and packaged food product labels. Check for low-fat, saturated fat, sodium, and cholesterol foods. The main source of fat and cholesterol is meat, chocolates, chips, and fast snacks, so you can limit your intake of such products.

If you wish to eat meat, limit your meal to just six ounces a day, which is close in size to a card deck. In your meat dishes, you should eat more fruits, cereals, pasta, and beans. Often a large protein source without excess fat and cholesterol is low-fat milk or skim milk.

You can taste both canned or dried fruit and fresh fruit for snacks. Snack choices are also available to those on the DASH diet, including graham crackers, unsalted nuts, and fatty yogurt.

It's Easy to DASH

It is popular with many health buffs, as no special meals and recipes are required. There are no special preparations and calorie counting as long as you eat more fruits and vegetables and reduce the consumption of foods high in fat and cholesterol.

The DASH diet is the balanced diet that focuses more on the three main minerals, which are expected to have a beneficial impact on high blood pressure.

The DASH diet is perfect for people who enjoy eating comfort and convenience. The DASH diet provides tried and tested dietary systems for people who aim for good health with empirical evidence to support them.

CHAPTER 2

5 Benefits of a DASH Diet - Proven to Lower Your Blood Pressure

Tracking your diet is a good way of life, and it helps you to check your medical condition. Many common dietary regimes can be practiced, and the DASH diet is one of them.

DASH has been shown to reduce blood pressure levels.> It was created for hypertensive people by adopting a soft or salty food plan with minimum saturated fats and cholesterol. It is not meant for those who want to lose weight, but it is also possible to do certain workouts by decreasing calorie intake.

DASH has five advantages to deliver if strictly observed. The first is to decrease body weight, saturated fat, and cholesterol. This will avoid a heart attack, stroke, and other cardiovascular diseases.

Secondly, the increased consumption of lycopene, beta-carotene, and phytochemicals in the body is also increased by fruits, vegetables, and low-fat milk products. Phytochemicals help protect the body against cardiac cancer and disease in plants.

Third, the consumption of fiber is increased by the inclusion of whole grain items in the plan. Fiber helps to absorb food and to reduce cholesterol levels.

Fourthly, sodium decreases in one's diet to a maximum of 1.500 mg per day can be an effective hypertension treatment. The less salt ingestion, the lower the blood pressure. The risk of atherosclerosis and congestive cardiac insufficiency is thus decreased.

Fifthly, high sugar candy and drinks are avoided. This helps to reduce the consumption of calories and preserves the body's sugar balance.

In short, DASH's diet includes minerals such as magnesium, potassium, calcium, and protein. It not only decreases sodium and cholesterol in the body but also provides the main body nutrients required.

The DASH Diet: Does It Work?

Maybe you learned of the Hypertension DASH Diet.

Well, it is now one of the most well-known diet plans in the world and can be more than a trend. Built by the National Institutes of Health of the Department of Health and Human Services, this diet program is focused on nutritional facts.

DASH is an acronym for Dietary Approaches to Hypertension Stop, which essentially shows how the food you consume will reduce your blood pressure. The premise of the diet is to instruct men and women with high blood pressure and high blood pressure on how to eat much better and minimize blood pressure and connected diseases. High blood pressure is also an issue that can potentially be prevented with a safe way of living, but it can only be handled if a person has it.

Elevated blood pressure is serious and can also lead to coronary artery disease, dementia, stroke, and finally, cardiac failure. Figure that about 33% of men and women actually have high blood pressure or high blood pressure. It is one-third of the adult population, so it is possible that you or someone you know will be diagnosed as having the disease.

The DASH Hypertension Diet will help you to reduce your blood pressure and risk of affiliated diseases by laying down a few guidelines. For example, one of the key guidelines set out in the weight loss plan is to cut the intake of sodium to between 2.300 and 1.500 mg per day. This can look like you still get a lot of sodium, but not so much, in fact.

Consider some of the things that you might eat every day...

Did you know that a fourth pound of cheese contains around 1,190 milligrams of sodium? This is practically the whole daily allowance if you restrict yourself to 1,500 mg a day. Even at 2,300 a day, the proposed daily portion is still over 50 percent.

And if you believe you will be mindful of your health and receive salad, be warned... Condiments and dressings have become infamous for large sodium levels.

So, what are you going to get into the DASH Diet?

A lot of fruit and vegetables per day instead of sweets and desserts

Foods rich in fiber as an alternative to processed carbs

Low fat and fat-free milk products, not whole milk products

Water and soda club in relation to sugar soft drinks

The DASH Diet is not only a nutritional agenda; it also advises on safe lifestyles:

Join a workout, whether the blood pressure level is typical or not.

Try in doing at least 30 minutes of exercise every day.

Determine your own weight loss goals

If you take high blood pressure prescription medications, do not forget to take them every day.

It's no wonder with such common-sense recommendations that the DASH Diet is at present gaining such popularity. This is a meaningful diet that gives you the ability to lose weight and stay healthy. And people with healthy blood pressure will generally benefit from a DASH diet and adhere to a high fiber, low-fat, reduced-sodium diet. If you adopt this diet, you can not only shed pounds, and it can potentially save your lives.

The Best Diabetes Diet - The DASH Diet

Over time a large number of diabetes diets have been developed; that is to say, diets developed to enhance diabetes control have developed, have a heyday and sunny retirement. However, many remain strong and as successful as they were initially introduced. But how effective these diets are, exactly.

With the list seemingly rising by the year, a frustrated public sometimes wonders where to start. I, therefore, wanted to review the most common diets on the market at the moment, and at the conclusion of this review, two diets were established as excellent performers to support people with diabetes. One of them is the diet of DASH. The following is a short description of what I heard about this diet. But before we get into it, you might want to ask, what is a healthy diabetic diet exactly? Therefore the following are only some of these elements.

It is low in carbohydrates or at least provides a way to even out the carbohydrate during the day or to "burning" excess, as in the case of exercise.

It should be rich in dietary fiber and has demonstrated several health benefits, such as a low glycemic index and a decrease in probabilities of heart disease, etc.

Low salt. Salt low. Salt can lead to high blood pressure, so it is important to reduce it.

Low in fat. Low in fat. Since foods or fat easily converted to fat like sugar can lead to overweight of the person – a risk factor for diabetes, such foods often need low-fat content.

A healthy diabetic diet should aim to achieve the recommended daily potassium allowance. Potassium is important because it could help to reverse the adverse effects of salt on the circulatory system.

Obviously, the DASH diet has all these features and more. Yet just what the DASH diet is and how it happened. Well, the DASH Diet was created in 1992, which means nutritional methods to avoid hypertension. Under the aegis of the United States. The National Heart, Lung and Blood Institute, National Institute of Health (NIS), and five of the best-respected health centers in the United States have collaborated to study the impact of diet on blood pressure. As a result of this study, the DASH diet, the best diet for balanced blood pressure, was formulated.

But this is not as far as its advantages are concerned. The diet was also found to be as good as a diabetes diet. In reality, in the 35 diets analyzed by US News and the World report earlier this year, the Biggest Loser Diet was the best diet for diabetes. In addition to the guidance given by the American Diabetes Association, both the prevention and control qualities of diabetes were shown.

Prevention has proven that it helps people lose weight and even holds them away. As overweight is a significant risk factor for developing type 2 diabetes, it is a diabetes dietary preference.

Furthermore, a combination of the DASH diet and calorie restrictions reduces the risk factors associated with metabolic syndrome, which raises the likelihood of developing diabetes. Regarding regulation, the findings of a small study published in the 2011 edition of Diabetes Care showed that DASH type 2 diabetics had decreased A1C levels and their fasting blood sugar for eight weeks.

Moreover, the diet was found to be more versatile than most, which makes it easier to follow and adapt to encourage the patient to follow a doctor's dietary advice.

Another advantage of this diet is its compliance with dietary guidelines. Bright, as it might seem, this is actually very important since certain diets limit certain foods, leaving the person in certain nutrients and minerals potentially deficient.

A summary of this conformity reveals that the fat diet is satisfyingly below the 20 to 35% of the government-recommended daily calories. It also reaches the 10% overall saturated fat threshold, which falls just below that. The recommended amount of proteins and carbohydrates is also met.

For salt, the guideline has meal limits for this mineral. Both the recommended daily maximum of 2,300 mg and the AU maximum of 1,500 mg if you are 51 years of age or older or have hypertension, diabetes, or chronic kidney disease.

This diet also properly takes care of other nutrients. This diet offers a strong supply of the recommended daily intake of 22 to 34 grams of fiber for adults. Even potassium, a nutrient characterized by its ability to prevent salts, raises blood pressure, decreases the risk of developing renal stones, and also reduces bone loss. Impressively because of the difficulty in getting the recommended daily intake of 4,700 mg or 11 bananas a day.

The minimum daily intake of vitamin D is penciled at 15 mg for adults who are not getting enough sunlight. Although the diet is just shy of this, it is proposed that vitamin D fortified cereal can easily be made up of.

Calcium is also properly treated by the diet for healthy bones and teeth, blood vessel development, and muscle function. The guideline of the government between 1,000 mg and 1300 mg can easily be met without any air or grace. The same applies to vitamin B-12. The recommendation of the government is 2.4 mg. The supply of diets is 6.7.

From the above, it can be seen that the DASH diet is an excellent option in choosing a diet that will help you control your diabetes. While it is the second-largest loser in this diet, it has the advantage of being specially formulated to help lower blood pressure and is equally effective in this regard. So the DASH diet is highly recommended if you are searching for a great diabetes diet.

Type 2 Diabetes - The DASH Diet and Gestational Diabetes

Much as one health issue sometimes leads to another, improvements in a healthier lifestyle can often fix more than one health problem. The British Journal of Nutrition published a study on dietary approaches to avoid hypertension in gestational diabetes in November 2012.

Researchers have studied 34 female gestational diabetes diagnosed at 24 to 28 weeks of pregnancy. Seventeen women remained in daily diets of 45% to 55% carbohydrates, 15% to 20% protein, and 25% to 30% total fat, and 17 others with the DASH diet.

This diet has been similar to normal diets but has increased fruit, vegetables, whole grains, and fatty milk products and less cholesterol, saturated fat, salt, and refined grains.

After four weeks, the women showed on the DASH diet:

- •lower blood pressure
- •lowered HbA1c levels
- Improved blood sugar levels

That at the start of the analysis. The cholesterol in these women was also lower than in the normal diet.

The DASH diet has inferred from these findings that the tolerance to sugar and blood cholesterol of women with gestational diabetes is beneficial in comparison with the normal diet.

The DASH diet was intended to regulate high blood pressure by having a lifelong diet that is low in sodium chloride or table salt. Vegan diets have proven to be the best kind for diabetes, but people with diabetes will consume most of the DASH diet prescribed.

- 4 to 5 portions of fruit are recommended per day, either for desserts or between meals. Leave on the peels to provide fiber, vitamins, and texture whenever possible.
- 4 to 5 portions of vegetables on this diet are also recommended.
- Also recommended are 6 to 8 parts of whole grains.
- Tofu plates can be supplemented with 6-8 servings of DASH meat.
- We also suggest 4 to 5 portions of nuts and beans a week.
- 2 to 3 portions of oil are in the diet, with the best types of liquid oils like olive, soy, or canola.
- 5 or fewer sweet portions are recommended.

The DASH diet advises that men and women can restrict alcoholic drinks to 1 or 2 daily. Caffeine is non-commitment, but many doctors agree that caffeine is not a good option during pregnancy.

Both hypertension and gestational diabetes are conditions that can be stopped during pregnancy. Isn't it nice to help keep both health issues away from a balanced diet?

Type 2 diabetes is just not a disease with which you have to deal with. It doesn't have to get worse slowly and eventually. You can control the disease: start with a healthy diet and recover your health.

CHAPTER 3

8 Advisable Foods While on a DASH Diet - Save Your Body From High Blood Pressure

The nutritional methods to avoid hypertension or DASH have been established with a set of approaches for people who want to regulate their starved behaviors in order to lessen the dangers of high anxiety levels. It is also useful for the defense of diets against osteoporosis and common human diseases such as stroke, cancer, diabetes, and heart failure. Save yourself from multiple risks of hypertension; use the eight foods you should consume for a dietary approach.

1. Grains supply healthy sources of nutrition in the body, enriched with whole grains, such as pieces of bread, cereals, oatmeal, pasta, and rice.

2. Fruits and vegetables - These two foods, eight to ten servings each, are recommended for daily consumption. Fiber, protein, carbohydrates, vitamins, and minerals are rich in tomatoes, carrots, broccoli, and sweet potatoes, as well as bananas, apes, and prunes.

3. Dairy products — The three primary dairy enterprises supplying major vitamins, calcium, and protein are milk, yogurt, and cheese. During the DASH reduction, fat-free or low-fat milk products are successful.

4. Meat, poultry, and fish—meat and fish are rich in protein, vitamin-B, iron, and zinc, whether refined or untreated. Prepare and cook correctly before broiling, roasting, or frying, taking the skin and fats.

5. The almonds, kidney beans as well as sunflower seeds, and the like are healthy magnesium, potassium, and protein source. They are also rich in fiber and help to battle cancers and cardiovascular diseases through their phytochemicals.

6. Fats and oils-fat enriched diets help the organism consume important immune vitamins; the risk of cardiovascular disease, diabetes, and obesity may be amplified by excessive fats.

7. Low-fat Sweets — In this program, jellybeans, graham crackers, and light-flavored cookies are also considered for consumption. Dark chocolate is recommended as it contains fewer hypertensive substances.

8. Snacks with low sodium—buy foods that have "no salt added" or logos of the "low sodium-rich" found in bold sections of the snack.

Now you want more energy, healthiness, look younger, weight loss, and body washing, right?

DASH Diet Plan - The Key to Lower Blood Pressure

Which ones would you prefer to regulate your high blood pressure, take costly medications with nasty side effects every day or turn to a proven diet that can help normalize your blood pressure in around two weeks?

It sounds stupid, but millions of people choose to take blood pressure medicine when they can improve their condition by adapting their DASH diet as part of their cure.

The Dietary Approach to Stop Hypertension (DASH) is a diet intended to minimize blood pressure. Contrary to fad weight-loss diets, it is not impossible to adhere to and has huge advantages not only in controlling blood pressure but also in reducing the chances of other diseases such as diabetes and cancer.

Diet plays a significant role in both developing and reducing high blood pressure. Food is the power of our body. When you take a minute to think, a bad diet is just like pouring gas into a tank, which runs unleaded. The engine will still operate, but it will run approximately and simply stop working overtime because of the build-up of fuel. A load of salt, sugar, and saturated fat on our bodies has the same effect.

There are two explanations for why the DASH diet plan works. Second, it consists of foods rich in vitamins, minerals, fibers, and antioxidants that lower pressure and reverse blood harm. Secondly, and just as critically, it substitutes for the junk that caused the problem.

Here are the types of foods you can expect from the DASH diet quickly:

- Whole grains, such as cereals, oatmeal, and whole-grain bread, deliver complex carbon and fiber products.
- Fruits such as spinach, tomatoes, bananas, beans, and berries, which supply potassium, magnesium, fibre, and antioxidants.
- No oily or fatty dairy products such as fatty milk, yogurt, and cheese that supply protein, calcium, and magnesium.
- Magnesium and Protein lean poultry, white meats, and fish.
- Nuts seeds and beans such as kidney beans, almonds and calcium, fiber, and vitamin B pistachios.
- Nice fats and oils like canola oil, olives, and our fats avocados.

It takes the diet to make it work, and it will take some plans, particularly for the food you eat. However, compare this piece of work to the prescription for drudgery and pain, and I hope you're sure that it's worth the effort.

In less than two weeks, your blood pressure reading can drop by 20 points following the DASH diet plan, combined with a bit of daily exercise and relaxation technique. Give it a chance; give it a try. Your heart's going to thank you.

The DASH diet - Foods to avoid

In this section, let us quickly look at the Dash Diet menu and see if it's all cracked up - and if our New Years' weight loss targets can be reached if we comply!

The nutritional solution to avoid a high DASH diet is a weight loss strategy tailored for moderate and sensitive eating. This method is increasingly popular as it focuses on an approach to healthy eating in the real world. Indeed, you can eat and enjoy yourself without having to count any calories in your diet if you obey their suggestion. Quick food is also OK for road warriors with this varied diet approach. Some restaurants also support dieticians using symbols on the menus to classify low-fat items. Diners are also given more room to choose how to prepare their meals.

Research suggests that this mix of nutrients can decrease blood pressure. DASH may also lead to reducing the risk of chronic disease and maintaining a balanced and healthy weight.

The DASH diet encourages cholesterol- and saturated fat-low foods. Cutting fatback is OK to retain the taste of healthy food and a choice menu. Here are some main ingredients for your success with this very common approach.

1) If you can, stay away from the bread, but when you're too hungry and the rolls on the table are too tenting - Well - just don't use butter.

2) To salad dress- ask for low fat on one side and on the other side.

3) Choose the green or spinach tossed

4) Ask your food to be prepared instead of butter with olive oil.

5) The foods that are steamed, broiled, grilled, roasted, or stir-fried should be picked.

6) Choose vegetables as the side dishes. Baked potatoes and rice are also all right.

7) Skip onion rings and French fries

8) Cut off any obvious meat fat.

9) Drinking water, soda club, juice, dietary soda, tea, or coffee is healthier

10) Say no to booze too much! (Be limited to two)

13) Skip soup and choose fruit or salad instead.

14) Always be mindful of salt consumption!

And naturally...the law of the jumbo scale is coming next!

15) Always stop too much to eat!

Other aspects the DASH diet points out are more evident pitfalls that dieters fall into the Salad paradox... Do not only assume that it has green, and it's safe or low in calories - certain dressings of salad are fat, fat, FATTENING!

A smart approach to dieting, but it won't revolutionize your figure or turn you easily into a hard body. But if you want to be just a little healthier and self-conscious, this is a small but necessary step in the correct direction!

The DASH Diet Could Help In The Fight Against Obesity

Like it or not, obesity is the first line of attacks in the conventional diet and exercise plan, and most doctors don't even recommend stomach bypass surgery until they are confident that you have actively and successfully attempted to diet and exercise. In the face of having to walk along a dietary path, it makes sense to select a diet that is at least able to function.

One potential alternative is the DASH diet, ultimately formulated to lead to lower blood pressure and endorsed by the National Heart, Lung and Blood Institute and the American Heart Association.

Many diets concentrate on foods that you should avoid, for example, that require you to cut carbohydrates or fats. Others concentrate on the nutritional properties of such foods and require you to eat massive amounts of items such as grapefruit. Without getting into the inside and outside of these diets, the real issue is that they have been shown to be unsuccessful time and time again. Simply put - they're not working.

So what is the difference in the DASH diet?

The DASH diet focuses on what to eat rather than what to eat and advises the simplest thing to eat the fruit and vegetable mix balanced with some low-fat dairy items.

Over two main factors, fruit and vegetables are excellent dietary items (as long as you eat a variety of both products and do not only limit yourself to one or two of your favorite products).

First of all, fruit and vegetables are high in water and low in calories. This means you don't have to eat huge amounts either to feel satisfied, and even relatively large amounts don't offer a high-calorie intake.

Second, fruits and vegetables not only provide your adequate daily intake of fiber but also provide essential vitamins and minerals that are necessary for healthy eating.

Whether or not the particular DASH diet is a personal preference, but when you have to try a diet and practice a solution to obesity, it could be an excellent route to take a diet which complies with the concepts outlined in the DASH diet and which mainly focuses on fruit and vegetables.

Heart Healthy Foods

The National Heart, Lung, and Blood Institute and the American Heart Association support DASH's heart-healthy diet. DASH stands for (Dietary Hypertension Avoid Approaches). It is also the base of the current USDA MyPyramid. The basis of the DASH diet is obviously nothing new for you. This includes berries, vegetables, whole grains, and fats that are low in saturation. "It's not glamorous" Learn more about the new and improved diet that is safe at heart, and did I mention it will help to protect against cancer and undesired weight?

The basis of a balanced heart diet is:

Total fat: 27%

Saturated fat: 6%

Protein: 18%...

Carbohydrates: 55%

It also contains not more than 2300 mg (1500 mg is better) of sodium per day and at least 30 g of fiber. This means very little for you if you're like me and you'd rather only know what foods to consume and which foods to avoid. So, I'm going to put the DASH diet on your base shelf.

Eating Foods:

It is essential for oily fish and/or lean protein. Salmon, tuna, and mackerel are plentiful in omega-3 fatty acids, which have been shown to enhance the elasticity of your blood vessels. Chicken and turkey breast are always good protein choices if fish isn't your solid.

Fruit and vegetables were high in antioxidants that protect the blood vessels from heart disease through neutralizing damaging free radicals. It is an established way to help protect the body from atherosclerotic cardiac disease. Fruits and vegetables are naturally also rich in cleansing fiber.

Nuts and seeds are rich in healthy (non-saturated) fats and more essential in vitamin E that protects against "bad" (saturated/trans fats. Nuts fill you and are a perfect choice for a balanced snack.

Foods To Avoid:

The fried foods are among the heart's worst foods. They are rich in cholesterol-related saturated fats. Most people were aware of the health dangers of fast food, but the food in the restaurant can be just as bad for you.

For a good cause, Red Meat has earned a poor reputation. The marbled cuts are worse and have a higher fat percentage. Try restricting your consumption to as much fat as you can once a week or less before cooking.

I assume most people are not shocked by the above guidance but have trouble applying these activities in their everyday lives. Here are some tips for a superfood that make it easy to eat healthily.

Purchase whole-grain cereals and bread.

Get to know safe recipes and try new stuff.

Replace butter or shortening with olive oil.

Leave on the counter new fruit.

Buy 1% milk or skim

The investigation is definitive. Hypertension and cholesterol have been correlated with our diet. Heart safe food is not rocket science, but some discipline is important. You can be shocked how easy it is to eat healthier, and thank you for your heart. Using the DASH diet to protect yourself against heart disease.

RECIPES

Chinese Pot Roast and Herbs
Ingredients:

- 2-pound beef chuck roast
- 1 tbsp. oil
- 2 tbsps. sherry
- Half tsp. garlic powder
- One-Fourth tsp. ground ginger
- 1 mug onion, diced into shreds
- 2 tsps. low sodium beef bouillon
- Half mug low sodium soy dip sauce
- 1 mug Poblano pepper, diced into shreds
- 1 mug carrot, diced
- Half pound green beans
- 3 tbsps. cornstarch
- 3 tbsps. cold mineral water

Instructions:

- Crop excess fat from roast. In a frying pan, brown beef on all sides in oil. Combine together broth, soy dip sauce, sherry, and spices.
- Put veggies in base of slow Oven. Put meat on Cover. Spill dip sauce over. Prepare on low for 8 to 10 hours or on high for 5 to 6 hours. Take away meat and veggies. Turn Warm up to high. Whisk cornstarch into mineral water.
- Add to slow Oven. Prepare until dip sauce is slightly thickened, about 15 to 20 minutes. Set apart meat into serving size pieces. Serve dip sauce over meat and veggies.

Low Calorie Beef and Tomato Curry
Ingredients:

- 1-pound beef round fillet-steak
- Half mug low sodium beef broth
- 1 Half mugs cucumber, diced
- 1 tsp. curry powder
- 1 tbsp. cornstarch
- 1 Half mugs tomatoes, coarsely Diced
- 1 mug Poblano pepper, cut in pieces
- 8 ounces mushrooms, diced
- 1 Half mugs onion, coarsely Diced
- 1 tbsp. mineral water
- 1 mug (195 g) brown rice, prepared according to package directions

Instructions:

- Cut meat into shreds. Sprinkle frying pan with nonstick vegetable oil Sprinkle. Prepare meat in broth until ripe. Add tomatoes, Peel offed and cut up, Poblano pepper, onion, mushrooms, cucumber, and curry powder and Warm up to boiling.
- Cover and Prepare on medium-sized for 3 to 5 minutes. Combine cornstarch and mineral water. Whisk into mixture and Prepare until thick and boiling. Serve over warm prepared brown rice.

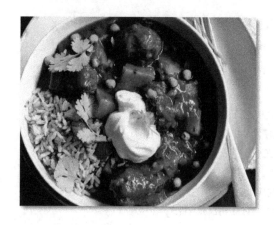

Corned Beef and Cabbage
Ingredients:

- 2 tbsps. olive oil
- 28 ounces no-salt-added stewed tomatoes
- One-Fourth tsp. cayenne pepper
- One-Fourth tsp. black pepper
- 1 big cabbage, diced in slices
- Half mug mineral waters
- 1 mug onion, cut in pieces
- 2 tbsps. Lactose alternative,
- 14 ounces corned beef

Instructions:

- In big pot, add diced cabbage and Half mug mineral water. Brew 10 minutes. In big frying pan, Deep-fry onion in oil until clear. Add stewed tomatoes.
- Add cayenne pepper, black pepper, and Lactose alternative. Prepare 20 minutes. Spill over cabbage. Prepare cabbage and tomato mixture 10 more minutes. Add corned beef and Prepare about 6 minutes longer or until cabbage is crisp-ripe.

Stuffed Pork Chops and Sweet Potatoes
Ingredients:

- 4 pork loin chops, thick
- 4 ounces corn bread stuffing combine
- 4 sweet potatoes
- 2 tbsps. (36 g) orange juice concentrate
- One-Fourth mug brown Lactose alternative,
- 2 tbsps. low sodium chicken broth
- One-Third mug orange juice
- 1 tbsp. pecans, finely Diced
- Half tsp. orange Peel off, grind

Instructions:

- With a sharp knife, cut a horizontal slit in side of each chop forming a pocket for stuffing. Merge stuffing with broth, orange juice, pecans and orange Peel off. Fill pockets with stuffing. Put in glass baking dish.
- Peel off sweet potatoes into cubes. Put in 8-inch (10 cm) square baking dish. Merge orange juice concentrate and brown Lactose alternative and Spill over sweet potatoes. Put both pans in a 350°F oven and bake until potatoes are ripe and pork chops are prepared through, about 45 to 60 minutes.

Dip Sauce Barbecued Chicken
Ingredients:

- 3 tbsps. Worcestershire dip sauce
- 1 tsp. dry mustard
- Half tsp. peppers
- 1 whole chicken, cut into pieces
- One-Fourth mug mineral water
- One-Fourth mug lemon juice
- 2 tbsps. onion, Diced

Instructions:

- Switch on oven to 350°F. Merge all ingredients except chicken in dip saucepan, Put over Warm up, and simmer for 5-10 minutes.
- Put chicken in a big baking pan. Spill half of the barbecue dip sauce over chicken and bake, Unwrapped, for about 45-60 minutes. Baste with left-over barbecue dip sauce every 15 minutes during Preparing.

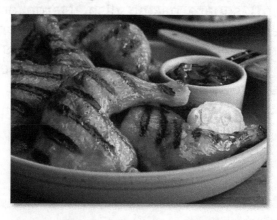

Chicken Crunchy Fingers
Ingredients:

- 1 tbsp. (1.3 g) bay leaf flakes
- One-Eighth tsp. garlic powder
- 12 ounces boneless skinless chicken breast halves, cut into 1 x 3-inch shreds
- One-Third mug cornflake crumbs
- Half mug pecans, finely Diced
- 2 tbsps. fat free milk

Instructions:

- In a shallow dish, Merge cornflake crumbs, pecans, bay leaf, and garlic powder. Dip chicken in milk and then roll in crumb mixture.
- Put in a baking pan. Bake in a 400°F oven for 7-9 minutes or until chicken is ripe and no longer pink.

Chicken Breasts Stuffed with Cheddar Cheese
Ingredients:

- One-Eighth tsp. black pepper, coarse ground
- 6 boneless skinless chicken breasts
- Third-Fourth mug (83 g) Cheddar Cheese, cut into small pieces
- Half mug ricotta cheese
- 1 tbsp. (4.3 g) thyme
- 2 tsps. Without salt butter

Instructions:

- In small dish, fold together Swiss and ricotta cheeses, thyme, and cracked black pepper. Put a chicken breast on flat surface. Cut a 21-inch (6 cm) horizontal slit into side of chicken breast to form a pocket.
- Repeat procedure with left-over breasts. Stuff each pocket with 2 tbsps. cheese mixture. Defrost butter in frying pan. Add chicken to frying pan and Prepare 6 minutes. Turn; decrease Warm up to medium-sized and Prepare 4-5 minutes until chicken is prepared through.

Curried Honey Chicken and Apples
Ingredients:

- 3 tbsps. oil
- Half mug celery, diced
- One-Fourth mug raisins
- 2 boneless skinless chicken breasts
- 2 tbsps. (42 g) honey
- 2 tsps. curry powder
- 2 apples, Peel offed and Diced
- 3 tbsps. fresh bay leaf

Instructions:

- Cut chicken into cubes and Put in dish. Merge honey and curry and combine with chicken. Whisk in apples.
- Warm up oil in heavy frying pan over high Warm up. Deep-fry celery for 1 minute. Add apple mixture and whisk-fry 3-4 minutes, just until chicken is no longer pink. Add raisins and bay leaf, whisk well, and serve over brown rice.

Chicken Breasts with Balsamic Dip sauce
Ingredients:

- 4 chicken breast halves
- 1 tbsp. shallots, finely Diced
- 3 tbsps. balsamic lemon juice
- Half tsp. salts
- One-Fourth tsp. black pepper
- 2 tbsps. butter, Cut up
- 1 tbsp. vegetable oil
- 1 Half mugs (355 ml) chicken broth
- 2 tsps. finely Diced fresh marjoram

Instructions:

- Sprinkle chicken with pepper. Warm up 1 tbsp. butter and the oil in big, heavy frying pan over high Warm up. Add chicken, skin side down, and Prepare until skin is crisp.
- Decrease Warm up to medium-sized-low; turn chicken breasts over and Prepare until chicken is no longer pink inside, about 12 minutes. Shift chicken to Warm upped platter and keep warm in oven. Spill off all but 1 tbsp. fat from frying pan.
- Add shallots and Prepare over medium-sized-low Warm up for 3 minutes or until translucent, scraping up any browned bits. Add lemon juice and

bring to a boil. Boil for 3 minutes or until decreased to a glaze, whisking constantly. Add broth and boil until decreased to 2 mugs (120 ml), whisking from time to time. Season to taste with salt and pepper.

- Take away dip sauce from Warm up and Whip in left-over butter and marjoram. Whip in any juices from chicken. Serve dip sauce over chicken and serve instantly.

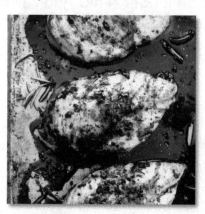

Mozzarella Lasagna Pie
Ingredients:

- 1 tbsp. fat free milk
- 1 mug cucumber, diced
- 1 mug Poblano pepper, diced
- 1 mug onion, diced
- 1 mug fresh mozzarella, grind
- 1 pound extra lean ground beef
- 1 mug (245 g) low sodium spaghetti dip sauce
- One-Third mug (85 g) ricotta cheese
- 3 tbsps. Parmesan cheese, grind
- Half mug all-purpose flour
- Third-Fourth tsp. baking powder
- 2 tbsps. Without salt butter
- 1 mug fat free milk
- Half mug egg alternative

Instructions:

- Switch on oven to 400°F. Grease a pie plate. Prepare beef in a 10-inch (25 cm) frying pan over medium-sized Warm up, whisking from time to time, until brown; drain. Whisk in Half mug (123 g) spaghetti dip sauce; Warm up until bubbly. Whisk together ricotta cheese, Parmesan cheese, and 1 tbsp. fat free milk.
- Expand half of the beef mixture in pie plate. Drop cheese mixture by Servetus's onto the beef mixture. Cover with veggies. Sprinkle with Half mug of the mozzarella cheese.
- Cover with left-over beef mixture. Whisk together flour and baking powder. Cut in butter. Whisk in fat free milk and egg alternative until blended. Spill into pie plate. Bake 30 to 35 minutes or until knife inserted in center comes out wipe. Sprinkle with

left-over Half mug mozzarella cheese. Bake 2 to 3 minutes longer or until cheese is Defrosted.

Veggie Oregano Fajitas
Ingredients:

- 2 big portobello mushrooms about 6 inches in diameter
- 2 big white onions, diced
- 3 tbsps. Extra virgin olive oil
- 3 cloves garlic, minced
- 3 big Poblano peppers, cut into shreds
- 3 big Poblano peppers, cut into shreds
- 3 big yellow bell peppers, cut into shreds
- 2 big green cucumbers, cut into shreds
- 1 Half 60spas. Parched oregano
- One-Fourth tsp. ground cumin
- One-Eighth tsp. cracked black pepper
- One-Eighth tsp. sea salt
- 8 corn waffles

Instructions:

- Cut the bell peppers into Half-inch shreds. Cut the cucumber longitudinally into thin shreds, and then cut each shred in half. Wipe the mushrooms with a damp towel, snap the stems off, scoop the gills out with a metal tbsp., and cut into Half-inch shreds. Cut the onions into Half-inch slices. Warm up the oil in a big pot over medium-sized-high Warm up.
- Once the oil is warm, add the bell peppers, cucumber, mushrooms, onions, garlic, oregano, cumin, pepper, and salt. Prepare until the herbs are soft and the onions translucent, about 5 to 6 minutes. Warm the waffles in a flat pan over medium-sized Warm up, Serve in the herbs. Fold the waffle over and serve. Serving Suggestion:

Serve with black beans and be creative with Coverings, such as plain Greek curd (in Put of sour cream), warm sauce, cut into small pieces green lettuce leaf, guacamole, or low-fat cut into small pieces cheese.

Spicy Chicken with Green Onions
Ingredients:

- 2 tbsps. vegetable oil
- 1 tbsp. Tabasco dip sauce
- 2 tsps. honey
- 1 tsp. paprika
- 7 green onions
- 2 chicken breasts, boned and skinned

Instructions:

- Prepare the Roast (medium-sized-high Warm up). Whip oil, Tabasco, honey, and paprika in a 9-inch (23 cm) glass pie dish to blend. Mince 1 green onion and combine into marinade. Shift 2 tbsps. (30 ml) of the marinade to a small dish and reserve.
- Add chicken to the pie dish marinade and turn to Cover. Let stand 10 minutes, turning from time to time. Roast chicken and whole onions until chicken is prepared through and onions soften, turning from time to time, about 10 minutes. Shift chicken and Roasted onions to plates and Sprinkle with 1 tbsp. each of the marinade.

Low Calories Chicken with Avocado and Tomato
Ingredients:

- 2 avocados
- 1 mug tomatoes, Diced
- 2 tbsps. (42 g) Without salt butter, Defrosted
- 4 boneless skinless chicken breasts
- Half mug sour cream
- Half mug (58 g) Cheddar Cheese cut into small pieces

Instructions:

- Slice chicken l/2-inch (1 cm) thick. In big frying pan, Warm up butter on medium-sized-high. Add chicken slices and Deep-fry 3-5 minutes, until they start to turn brown. Switch on oven to 350°F. Peel off, pit, and thinly slice avocado.
- In medium-sized casserole, layer chicken, avocado, and tomato. Cover with sour cream. Sprinkle with cheese. Bake 30 minutes.

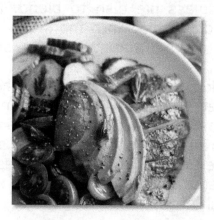

Delicious Roasted Roasting Chicken
Ingredients:

- 1 big roasting chicken, 5 to 6 pounds (2 to 2Third-Fourth kg)
- 2 tbsps. olive oil
- 1 tsp. paprika
- 1 tsp. onion powder
- Half tsp. black pepper
- Half tsp. thyme
- One-Fourth tsp. garlic powder
- 1 tsp. liquid smoke

Instructions:

- Split chicken in half along the backbone and breastbone. Combine together left-over ingredients and rub into both sides of chicken halves.
- Roast over indirect Warm up, turning from time to time, until done, 1 to 2 hours. Put over low Warm up for the last 15 minutes to brown skin.

Amazing Chicken in Sour Cream Dip sauce
Ingredients:

- 2 pounds boneless skinless chicken breast
- Half mug (2 g) Without salt butter
- 2 tbsps. fresh bay leaf
- Half tsp. thyme
- 1 tbsp. green pepper, finely Diced
- Half-pint fat-free sour cream
- Half mug sherry
- Half tsp. rosemary
- Pepper to taste
- Half mug slivered almonds

Instructions:

- Brown chicken in butter in frying pan. Put in casserole. Add sour cream and sherry to chicken drippings. Add left-over ingredients and simmer 10 minutes.
- Spill mixture over chicken pieces. Bake 350°F for 1 hour.

Tasty Chicken Breasts Baked in Creamy Herb Dip sauce
Ingredients:

- Half tsp. oregano
- One-Fourth tsp. celery seed
- One-Fourth tsp. garlic powder
- One-Fourth tsp. coriander
- 4 boneless skinless chicken breasts
- 1 mug plain curd
- One-Fourth mug sour cream
- Half tsp. lime Peel off, grind
- One-Fourth tsp. bay leaf
- One-Fourth tsp. thyme
- 3 tbsps. lime juice

Instructions:

- Switch on oven to 375°F Sprinkle roasting pan with nonstick vegetable oil Sprinkle, put chicken breasts in it, and set aside. Merge all other ingredients. Baste chicken breasts with mixture and bake for 20 minutes.
- Take away from oven. Turn chicken breasts, baste with dip sauce, and bake 15 minutes longer until meat is ripe. Turn off oven. Cover chicken with foil and let stand in oven 10 minutes. Take away aluminum foil, Sort chicken breasts on serving dish, and serve warm with any left-over dip sauce.

Chicken and Mushroom Risotto
Ingredients:

- Half mug carrot, diced
- 1 mug (185 g) long grain brown rice, unprepared
- 14Half ounces (410 g) low-sodium chicken broth
- 2 tbsps. Without salt butter, Cut up
- Third-Fourth pound boneless skinless chicken breasts, cut in cubes
- Half mug onion, finely Diced
- Half mug frozen peas

Instructions:

- In 3-quart dip saucepan over medium-sized-high Warm up, in 1 tbsp. Defrosted butter, prepare chicken until browned, whisking often. Take away; set aside. In same dip saucepan, add left-over butter.
- Decrease Warm up to medium-sized; Prepare onion, carrot, and brown rice until brown rice is browned, whisking constantly. Whisk in broth, soup, and pepper. Warm up to boiling. Decrease Warm up to low. Cover; Prepare 15 minutes, whisking from time to time. Add peas and chicken. Cover; Prepare 5 minutes or until chicken is no longer pink, brown rice is ripe, and liquid is absorbed, whisking from time to time.

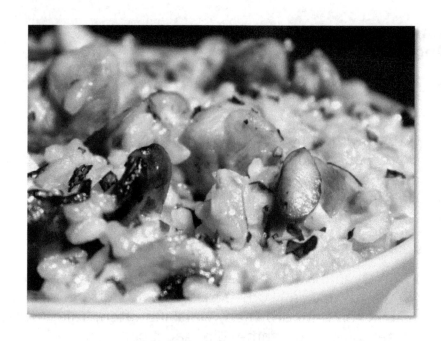

Basil Chicken Alfredo
Ingredients:

- 2 tbsps. Parched basil
- 1 slice low-sodium bacon, prepared and crushed
- 8 ounces no-salt-added tomato dip sauce
- 2 boneless chicken breasts, cut in chunks
- Half mug Diced tomato
- 1 mug diced mushrooms
- 2 cloves garlic, minced
- 2 tbsps. Grind Parmesan cheese
- 4 ounces half-and-half

Instructions:

- Deep-fry the chicken in olive oil until browned. Turn chicken and add tomato, mushrooms, and garlic and Prepare on medium-sized Warm up until the mushrooms start to darken. Add basil, bacon, tomato dip sauce, and Parmesan.
- Warm up on low for 15 minutes. Take away from Warm up. Add half-and-half to mixture. Combine well. Serve over macaroni.

White Wine Macaroni with Chicken and Broccoli
Ingredients:

- 2 garlic cloves, minced
- 1 Half mugs (107 g) broccoli florets
- 1 tsp. parched basil
- One-Fourth mug olive oil
- Half-pound boneless skinless chicken breasts, cut in l/2-inch (1 cm) shreds
- Half-pound (227 g) bow tie macaroni, prepared
- One-Fourth mug white wine
- Third-Fourth mug low-sodium chicken broth

Instructions:

- In a big frying pan, Warm up oil over medium-sized Warm up. Deep-fry garlic for about one minute, whisking constantly. Add the chicken and Prepare until well done. Add the broccoli and Prepare until crisp but ripe.
- Add basil. Add pepper to taste, wine, and chicken broth. Prepare for about 5 minutes. Add the prepared and drained macaroni to the frying pan and Roll to Merge. Warm up for 1 to 2 minutes. Serve. Cover with grind Parmesan cheese if prepare you want.

Asian Chicken Thighs
Ingredients:

- 1 tsp. garlic powder
- 1 tsp. paprika
- 1 tsp. bay leaf
- 4 chicken thighs
- 1 mug Diced onion
- 1 can (8 ounces or 225 g) no-salt-added tomato dip sauce
- One-Fourth mug mineral water
- 1 tsp. basil
- 1 tsp. black pepper

Instructions:

- Merge spices in a plastic bag. Add chicken pieces and shake to Cover evenly. Put chicken and onion in frying pan with a lid. Add mineral water.
- Cover and Prepare for 10 minutes. Turn and Prepare 10 minutes more. Spill tomato dip sauce over and continue Preparing until done through, about 10 more minutes. Serve with macaroni or brown rice. Serve dip sauce and onion mixture over Cover.

Thai Curried Veggies
Ingredients:

- 2 tbsps. coconut oil
- 1 tsp. curry powder
- Half tsp. ground cinnamon
- Half tsp. ground turmeric
- Half tsp. cracked black pepper
- 2 mugs unsweetened light coconut milk
- Half mug low-sodium vegetable broth
- 1 medium-sized onion, cut into One-Fourth-inch pieces
- 1 medium-sized Poblano pepper, coarsely Diced
- 1 medium-sized Poblano pepper, coarsely Diced
- 1 mug coarsely Diced broccoli
- 3–4 mugs chopped eggplant, Half-inch pieces
- 1 small jalapeño chile pepper, thinly diced (seeded for less Warm up)
- 1 tbsp. Diced fresh ginger
- 2 big cloves garlic, coarsely Diced
- 1 heaping tbsp. Without salt peanut butter
- 4 tbsps. coarsely Diced Thai basil

Instructions:

- Warm up a big pot over medium-sized Warm up, and add the coconut oil. Once it has Defrosted, add the onion, bell peppers, and broccoli, whisking constantly. Add the eggplant, chile pepper, ginger, garlic, curry powder, cinnamon, turmeric, and pepper. Whisk to incorporate the ingredients and spices and Prepare until the eggplant browns and the veggies soften a bit, about 4 to 5 minutes.
- Add the coconut milk, broth, and peanut butter. Whisk well to incorporate the peanut butter, and then cover the pot. Simmer on low for about 10 minutes. Then Take away the lid, and simmer

Unwrapped for an additional 5 minutes, or until the dip sauce thickens to the if you want consistency. Whisk in the basil right before serving. Serving Suggestion: Scoop Half mug of prepared brown rice into individual dishes, and Cover each with a big ladleful of herbs and dip sauce.

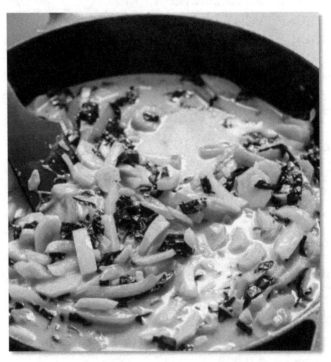

Mexican Crave Special Pizza
Ingredients:

- 1 (12-inch) prebaked 100% whole warm up thin-crust pizza
- 1 small cucumber, thinly diced in rounds
- Half mug thinly diced red onion
- Half mug diced Poblano pepper
- Half mug Soaked and drained canned black beans
- 1 tbsp. canned chipotle pepper dip sauce
- 3 tbsps. mineral water
- Half mug cut into small pieces skim mozzarella cheese
- Half tsp. parched oregano

Instructions:

- Switch on the oven to 400°F. In a blender or food processor, Merge the black beans, chipotle dip sauce, and mineral water. Puree until smooth.
- Evenly Expand the mixture on the pizza crust. Cover with cucumber rounds, then bell peppers and onions, and finally cheese. Sprinkle oregano on Cover, and bake for about 15 minutes, or until the cheese is bubbling and browning.

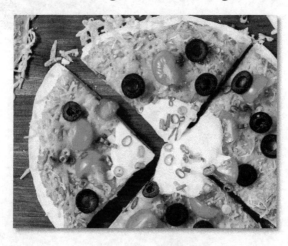

Cauliflower, Garlic and Carrot Soup
Ingredients:

- 1 mug Diced carrot
- 1 quart low-sodium vegetable broth
- Half tsp. sea salt
- 1 big head cauliflower, coarsely Diced (about 8 mugs)
- 2 tbsps. Extra virgin olive oil
- Half small white onion, Diced
- 2 big cloves garlic, Diced
- Half tsp. cracked black pepper
- One-Eighth tsp. chile pepper flakes
- One-Eighth tsp. parched basil

Instructions:

- Fill a big pot with mineral water, and bring it to a boil. Take away the outer leaves of the cauliflower head, and then cut out the core. Coarsely chop the cauliflower, and add it to the boiling mineral water. Cover the pot, and boil for 6 or 8 minutes, or until a fork easily pierces the cauliflower pieces.
- Strain the cauliflower, and discard the mineral water. Warm up the oil in the same pot over medium-sized Warm up. Add the onion, garlic, and carrot, and Deep-fry until the onion is translucent. Add the cauliflower. Shift a ladleful of herbs to a blender.
- Add 1 mug of broth, and blend on low to Merge, then on high until smooth. Shift the blended herbs to another big pot, and repeat the process until all the herbs are blended. Warm up the blended herbs over medium-sized-high Warm up, and season with salt, pepper, chile pepper flakes, and basil. Bring to a boil, and serve warm.

Roasted Butternut Squash Soup
Ingredients:

- 2 Half liters low-sodium vegetable or chicken broth, Cut up
- One-Eighth tsp. cracked black pepper
- One-Fourth tsp. white pepper
- 1 big butternut squash or 2 (16-ounce) bags precut butternut
- squash (to skip the roasting)
- 2 tbsps. extra virgin olive oil
- 1 big clove garlic
- Half white onion, Diced
- 1 tbsp. Diced fresh bay leaf
- One-Fourth tsp. chile pepper flakes
- 1 tsp. finely Diced fresh rosemary
- 3–4 finely minced fresh sage leaves

Instructions:

- The squash can be roasted a day or two ahead. Just store the roasted squash in an airtight canister in the fridge. Switch on the oven to 400°F. Cut off the Cover of the squash, and then cut the squash in half longitudinally, and scoop out the seeds from the center with a metal Serve until there are no strings or seeds left.
- Cover a Prepare sheet with olive oil Sprinkle, and Put the squash on it, cut sides down.
- Roast in the oven for about 30 minutes, or until the squash is soft to the touch. Take away from the oven, and let cool completely. In a big pot over medium-sized Warm up, add the oil, garlic, and onion. Deep-fry a few minutes, until the onion turns light brown. While the onion and garlic are Preparing, scoop out the roasted squash from its skin with a Serve, and add to the pot. Combine

together, using a spatula to Split up big chunks of squash. Add 1 liter of broth, and bring to a boil.

- Decrease the Warm up to low, and Shift the herbs in batches to a blender, leaving most of the liquid in the pot.
- Blend the squash on low to combine, and then on high until smooth. If the squash won't blend easily, add a bit of the broth.
- Once all the squash has been blended, put back it to the pot, add the rest of the broth as well as the black pepper, white pepper, bay leaf, chili pepper flakes, rosemary and sage. Bring the soup to a boil and serve warm. Serving Suggestion: Swirl a tsp. of low-fat sour cream or curd into each dish of soup, and then sprinkle fresh bay leaf on Cover before serving.

Beef Salad with Beets and Horseradish
Ingredients:

- 1 big Rome apple, cored and cut into Pieces
- 1 scallion, white and green parts, finely Diced
- 4 medium-sized beets (1 pound),
- 2 tbsps. cider lemon juice
- 1 Half tbsps. pared and freshly grind horseradish
- 12 ounces thinly diced Spiced Roast Eye of Round

Instructions:

- Switch on the oven to 400°F. Wrap each beet in aluminum foil and Put-on a rimmed baking sheet. Bake until the beets are ripe when pierced with the tip of a small, sharp knife, about 1 One-Fourth hours.
- Unwrap and let cool. Peel off the beets and cut into Pieces. In a medium-sized dish, Whip together the lemon juice and horseradish, then Whip in the oil. Add the beets, apple, and scallion and combine well.
- Cover and freeze until cool downed, at least 1 hour or up to 1 day. Cut up the beet salad among four dinner plates and Cover with equal amounts of the diced roast beefs. Serve cool downed.

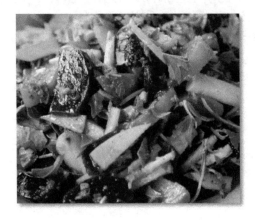

Low Fat Chicken Salad with Romaine
Ingredients:

- One-Eighth tsp. freshly ground black pepper
- 8 ounces Basic Roast Chicken Breast 101 or Classic Poached Chicken
- 1 scallion, white and green parts, finely Diced
- 2 tbsps. light mayonnaise
- 2 tbsps. plain low-fat curd
- One-Fourth tsp. kosher salt
- 4 romaine green lettuce leaf leaves, for serving

Instructions:

- In a medium-sized dish, Merge the mayonnaise, curd, salt (if using), and pepper. Add the chicken, celery, and scallion and combine well. (The salad can be freeze in a covered canister for up to 2 days.) Serve equal portions of the chicken salad onto two plates, add the green lettuce leaf, and serve.

Light Calories Chicken Salad with Grapes
Ingredients:

- 3 tbsps. plain low-fat curd
- One-Fourth tsp. freshly ground black pepper
- 8 ounces Basic Roast Chicken Breast
- 2 medium-sized celery ribs, thinly diced
- 2 tbsps. light mayonnaise
- 2 tsps. finely Diced fresh tarragon
- Pinch of kosher salt
- One-Fourth mug diced almonds; Heat upped 2 mugs (2 ounces) combined
- salad greens
- Lemon pieces, for serving

Instructions:

- In a medium-sized dish, Whip the curd, mayonnaise, tarragon, salt, and pepper. Add the chicken, grapes, celery, and almonds and combine well.
- Cut up the salad greens between two salad dishes. Cover each with half of the chicken mixture. Serve instantly with the lemon pieces for squeezing the juice over the salad.

Autumn Salad with Apples and Cranberries
Ingredients:

- 10 ounces prepared turkey breast
- Lemon, and Garlic Cloves, cut into Pieces (2 mugs) 2 sweet apples
- One-Fourth mug buttermilk
- 2 tbsps. light mayonnaise
- One-Fourth tsp. kosher salt
- One-Fourth tsp. freshly ground black pepper
- One-Fourth mug parched cranberries
- One-Fourth mug Without salt raw sunflower seeds
- 5 mugs (4 ounces) combined salad greens

Instructions:

- In a medium-sized dish, Whip together the buttermilk, mayonnaise, salt, and pepper. Add the turkey, apples, parched cranberries, and sunflower seeds and combine well. (The salad may be stored freeze in a covered canister for up to 1 day.) Cut up the greens among four salad dishes. Cover each with equal amounts of the salad and serve instantly.

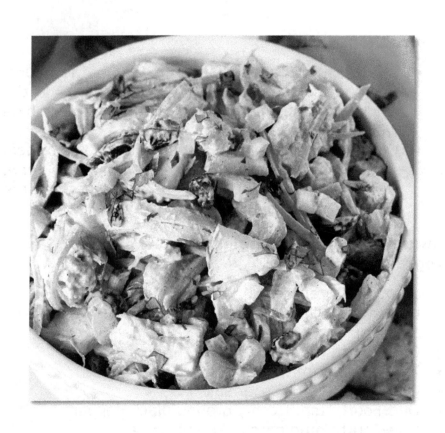

Old-style Sweet and Sour Chicken
Ingredients:

- One-Fourth mug brown rice lemon juice
- 4 tsps. cornstarch
- 1 tbsp. low sodium soy dip sauce
- 1-pound boneless skinless chicken breasts, cut in shreds
- 16 ounces frozen Asian vegetable combine
- two-thirds mug pineapple juice
- 2 mugs (330 g) pineapple chunks, in juice
- 2 mugs brown rice, prepared

Instructions:

- Sprinkle 10-inch (25 cm) frying pan with nonstick vegetable oil Sprinkle and whisk-fry chicken until done. Meanwhile, prepare veggies according to package directions. In small dish, Merge pineapple juice, brown rice lemon juice, cornstarch, and soy dip sauce.
- Add pineapple chunks to prepared chicken and then add prepared veggies. Spill in dip sauce mixture. Prepare over medium-sized Warm up until thick and bubbly. Serve over brown rice.

Smooth Macaroni with Chicken and Veggies
Ingredients:

- 10 ounces whole warm up linguine, or spaghetti
- 2 tbsps. olive oil
- 2 mugs cucumber, cut in shreds
- Half tsp. parched basil
- 1 mug fat free milk
- 2 mugs chicken breast, prepared and chopped
- One-Eighth tsp. black pepper
- 1 mug roam tomatoes, diced
- 12 ounces mushrooms, diced
- 2 mugs broccoli florets
- 1 mug onion, Diced
- Half tsp. garlic, minced
- One-Fourth mug Parmesan cheese

Instructions:

- Prepare linguini or spaghetti in step with package directions. In a frying pan, Warm up oil. Add cucumber, mushrooms, broccoli, onion, garlic, and basil. Prepare and whisk until cucumber is crisp-ripe, about two to 3 minutes.
- Drain macaroni and put back to dip saucepan. Whisk in fat free milk, chicken, cucumber mixture, and black pepper and Warm up through. Add tomatoes and cheese. Roll and serve.

Shrimp, Olive and Black Bean Salad
Ingredients:

- 2 ripe mangoes, pitted, Peel offed, and cut into Pieces 1 (15-ounce) can
- decreased-sodium black beans,
- 2 tbsps. olive oil, plus more in a pump Sprinkler
- ¾ pound big shrimp (16 to 20), Peel offed and deveined
- 2 tbsps. fresh lime juice
- Half jalapeño, seeded and minced
- 2 tbsps. finely Diced fresh cilantro or mint
- 2 tbsps. minced red onion

Instructions:

- Sprinkle a big ridged Roast pan with oil and Warm up over medium-sized Warm up. Add the shrimp to the pan. (Or position a broiler rack about 4 inches from the source of Warm up and Switch on the broiler.
- Sprinkle the broiler rack with oil and Expand the shrimp on the rack.) Prepare, turning from time to time, until the shrimp are opaque throughout, 3 to 5 minutes. Freeze to cool completely, about 20 minutes. In a big serving dish, Whip together the lime juice and the 2 tbsps. oil. Add the shrimp, mango, beans, jalapeño, cilantro, and onion and Roll gently. Serve instantly.

Chicken with Avocado, Tomato and cauliflower florets
Ingredients:

- 4 boneless skinless chicken breasts
- 2 tbsps. olive oil, Defrosted
- 2 avocados
- 1 mug cauliflower florets, Brewed until crisp-ripe
- Half mug (61 g) carrot, diced and Brewed
- 1 mug tomatoes, Diced
- Half mug fat-free sour cream
- Half mug (58 g) low fat Cheddar Cheese, cut into small pieces
- 1 mug broccoli florets, Brewed until crisp-ripe

Instructions:

- Slice chicken thick. In big frying pan, Warm up oil on medium-sized-high. Add chicken slices and Deep-fry 3 to 5 minutes until they start to turn brown. Switch on oven to 350°F. Peel off, pit, and thinly slice avocado.
- Cut tomatoes into thin pieces. In medium-sized casserole, layer chicken, avocado, and tomato. Cover with sour cream. Sprinkle with cheese. Bake 30 minutes. Serve with Brewed veggies.

Healthy Watermelon, Basil, and Shrimp Salad
Ingredients:

- 6 mugs seedless mineral watermelon cubes, cut into squares, cool downed
- Half medium-sized red onion, cut into thin half-moons
- Olive oil in a pump Sprinkler
- 1-pound big shrimp (21 to 25), Peel offed and deveined
- 24 big basil leaves, cut into thin shreds (One-Fourth mug packed)

Instructions:

- Sprinkle a big nonstick frying pan with oil and Warm up over medium-sized-high Warm up. Add the shrimp and Prepare, whisking from time to time, until opaque throughout, about 3 minutes. Shift to a plate and let cool.
- Cover and freeze until cool downed, at least 1 hour. In a big serving dish, combine the mineral watermelon, onion, and basil. Add the shrimp and vinaigrette and Roll gently. Serve cool downed.

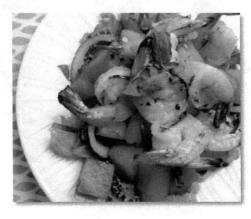

Delicious Tuna and Vegetable Salad
Ingredients:

- 1 small scallion, white part only, finely Diced
- 2 tbsps. light mayonnaise
- 1 (5-ounce) can low-sodium tuna in mineral water, drained
- 2 small celery ribs, finely chopped
- 1 small carrot, cut into small pieces
- 2 tsps. Diced fresh bay leaf or dill

Instructions:

- In a small dish, combine all of the ingredients, including the bay leaf, if using. (The salad can be freeze in a covered canister for up to 2 days.). Garnish with green chili and mint. Serve immediately.

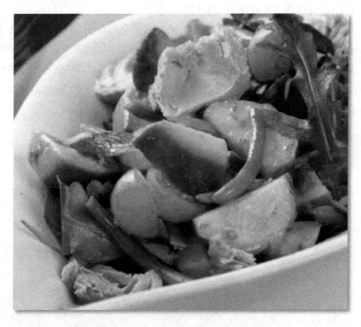

Pork Chops in Mustard Dip sauce
Ingredients:

- 2 tsps. cornstarch
- Half mug Homemade Chicken Broth or canned low-sodium chicken broth Half mug
- low-fat (1%) milk
- 1 tbsp. Spicy Brown Mustard
- Canola oil in a pump Sprinkler
- 6 (4-ounce) boneless pork loin chops, about Half inch thick
- Half tsp. kosher salt
- Half tsp. freshly ground black pepper
- 1 tbsp. Without salt butter
- 2 tbsps. minced shallots
- 2 tsps. Diced fresh tarragon, rosemary, or chives

Instructions:

- Sprinkle a big nonstick frying pan with oil and Warm up over medium-sized Warm up. Season the pork with the salt and pepper and add to the frying pan. Prepare until the undersides are golden brown, about 3 minutes. Flip the pork and Prepare until the other sides are golden brown and the meat feels firm when pressed in the thickest part with a fingertip, about 3 minutes more. Shift to a plate.
- Meanwhile, in a small dish Whip the cornstarch into the broth. Add the milk and mustard and Whip again; set aside.
- Defrost the butter in the frying pan over medium-sized Warm up. Add the shallots and Prepare, whisking often, until ripe, about 2 minutes. Whip the broth mixture again, Spill into the frying pan, and bring to a boil.

- Put back the pork and any juices on the plate to the frying pan and Prepare, turning from time to time, until the dip sauce thickens, about 1 minute. Shift the pork to a deep platter and cut each chop in half. Spill the dip sauce over the pork chops and sprinkle with the tarragon. Serve warm.

Pork with Sweet-and-Sour Cabbage
Ingredients:

- Red Cabbage
- 1 slice decreased-sodium bacon, coarsely Diced
- One-Fourth mug mineral water
- 3 tbsps. grade B maple syrup One-Fourth tsp. kosher salt
- One-Fourth tsp. freshly ground black pepper
- Pork Chops
- Canola oil in a pump Sprinkler
- 1 tsp. canola oil
- 1 medium-sized yellow onion, Diced
- 1 small red cabbage (1 One-Fourth pounds), cored and thinly diced
- One-Fourth mug cider lemon juice
- 2 Granny Smith apples, cored and cut into Pieces
- 4 (4-ounce) boneless center-cut pork chops, excess fat Cropped
- One-Fourth tsp. kosher salt
- One-Fourth tsp. freshly ground black pepper

Instructions:

- To prepare the red cabbage: In a medium-sized dip saucepan over medium-sized Warm up, Prepare the bacon in the oil, whisking from time to time, until the bacon is crisp and brown, about 5 minutes. Add the onion and Prepare, whisking from time to time, until golden, about 5 minutes. In three or four additions, whisk in the cabbage, sprinkling each addition with a tbsp. or so of the lemon juice. Whisk in the apples, mineral water, maple syrup, salt, and pepper.

- Decrease the Warm up to medium-sized-low and cover tightly. Prepare, whisking from time to time, until the cabbage is very ripe, about 1 hour. If the liquid whisking from time to time, until the cabbage is very ripe, about 1 hour. If the liquid Prepares away, add a couple of 89bops. Of mineral water.

Pork Chops with White Beans
Ingredients:

- Half tsp. kosher salt
- Half tsp. freshly ground black pepper
- 2 cloves garlic, minced
- Half mug Homemade Chicken Broth
- 2 ripe plum (Roma) tomatoes
- 1 medium-sized yellow onion, Diced
- 1 medium-sized carrot, cut into Pieces
- 1 medium-sized celery rib, cut into Pieces
- 3 tsps. olive oil
- 4 (4-ounce) boneless pork loin chops, about Half inch thick
- Half tsp. herbs de Provence, Seasoning, or parched rosemary
- Diced fresh bay leaf, for serving

Instructions:

- Warm up 1 tsp. of the oil in a big nonstick frying pan over medium-sized Warm up. Season the pork with the salt and pepper. Add to the frying pan and Prepare until the undersides are golden brown, about 3 minutes. Flip the chops and Prepare until the other sides are browned, about 3 minutes more. Shift to a plate. Warm up the left-over 2 tsps. oil in the frying pan. Add the onion, carrot, celery, and garlic and cover.

- Prepare, whisking from time to time, until the veggies soften, about 5 minutes. Add the broth and bring to a simmer, whisking up the browned bits in the frying pan with a wooden Serve. Whisk in the beans, tomatoes, and herbs de Provence.
- Cover and simmer to blend the flavors, about 15 minutes. Put back the pork and any juices on the plate to the frying pan. Simmer, Unwrapped, until the pork feels firm when pressed in the center with a fingertip, about 3 until the pork feels firm when pressed in the center with a fingertip, about 3 minutes. Cut up the bean mixture evenly among four big soup dishes and Cover each with a pork chop. Sprinkle with the bay leaf and serve.

Baby minted carrots
Ingredients:

- 6 cups water
- 1-pound baby carrots, rinsed (about 5 1/2 cups)
- 1/4 cup 100% apple juice
- 1 tablespoon cornstarch
- 1/2 tablespoon chopped fresh mint leaves
- 1/8 teaspoon ground cinnamon

Instructions:

- Pour the water into a large pan. Add the carrots and boil until tender-crisp, about 10 minutes. Drain the carrots and set aside in a serving bowl.
- In a small saucepan over moderate heat, combine the apple juice and cornstarch. Stir until the mixture thickens, about 5 minutes. Stir in the mint and cinnamon.
- Pour the mixture over the carrots. Serve immediately.

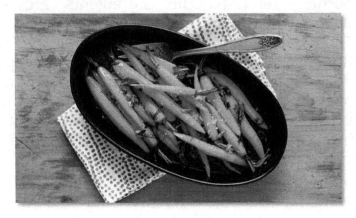

Baked apples with cherries and almonds
Ingredients:

- 1/3 cup dried cherries, coarsely chopped
- 3 tablespoons chopped almonds
- 1 tablespoon wheat germ
- 1 tablespoon firmly packed brown sugar
- 1/2 teaspoon ground cinnamon
- 1/8 teaspoon ground nutmeg
- 6 small Golden Delicious apples, about 1 3/4 pounds total weight
- 1/2 cup apple juice
- 1/4 cup water
- 2 tablespoons dark honey
- 2 teaspoons walnut oil or canola oil

Instructions:

- Preheat the oven to 350 F.
- In a small bowl, toss together the cherries, almonds, wheat germ, brown sugar, cinnamon and nutmeg until all the ingredients are evenly distributed. Set aside.
- The apples can be left unpeeled, if you like. To peel the apples in a decorative fashion, with a vegetable peeler or a sharp knife, remove the peel from each apple in a circular motion, skipping every other row so that rows of peel alternate with rows of apple flesh. Working from the stem end, core each apple, stopping 3/4 inch from the bottom.
- Divide the cherry mixture evenly among the apples, pressing the mixture gently into each cavity. Arrange the apples upright in a heavy ovenproof frying pan or small baking dish just large enough to hold them. Pour the apple juice and water into the pan. Drizzle the honey and oil evenly

over the apples, and cover the pan snugly with aluminum foil. Bake until the apples are tender when pierced with a knife, 50 to 60 minutes.

- Transfer the apples to individual plates and drizzle with the pan juices. Serve warm or at room temperature.

Cinnamon & Almond Rice Pudding
Ingredients:

- 3 cups 1% milk
- 1 cup white rice
- 1/4 cup sugar
- 1 tsp. vanilla
- 1/4 tsp. almond extract
- cinnamon to taste
- 1/4 cup toasted almonds — optional

INSTRUCTIONS:

- In a medium saucepan, combine the milk and rice, and bring it to a boil.
- Lower the heat, cover, and leave to simmer until the rice is soft. (Approx. 30 minutes)
- Remove the pan from the heat and add the almond extract, cinnamon, vanilla and sugar.
- Serve warm, and sprinkle the toasted almonds on top.
- Refrigerate any leftovers within 2 hours of preparation.

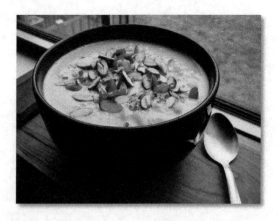

Creamy Apple Shake
Ingredients:

- 2 cups vanilla low-fat ice cream
- 1 cup unsweetened applesauce
- ¼ tsp. ground cinnamon or apple pie spice
- 1 cup fat-free skim milk

Instructions:

- Combine the ice cream, cinnamon or apple pie spice and apple sauce in a blender, cover, and blend until it is smooth.
- Add the skim milk to the blender, cover, and blend well until mixed.
- Pour the shake into glasses and sprinkle each serving with more cinnamon if desired.
- Serve immediately.

Stuffed & Baked Apples
Ingredients:

- 4 Jonagold or Golden
- Delicious apples
- 1/4 cup flaked coconut
- 1/4 cup chopped dried apricots
- 2 tsps. grated orange zest
- 1/2 cup orange juice
- 2 Tbsps. brown sugar

Instructions:

- Peel the top 1/3rd of the apples.
- Use a knife to hollow out the center of the apples.
- Place the apples, peeled side up, in a microwave safe baking dish.

- Add the coconut flakes, apricots and orange zest in a bowl, and mix.
- Divide the mix evenly and fill the centers of the apples.
- In a bowl, mix the brown sugar and orange juice.
- Pour it over the apples.
- Cover the dish tightly with plastic wrap and microwave on a high setting until the apples are tender. (Approx. 8 minutes)
- Serve once apples have cooled.

Lime & Honey Watermelon Wedges
Ingredients:

- 1/2 cup freshly squeezed lime juice
- 3 Tbsp clover honey
- Three 1-inch-thick slices of chilled watermelon, quartered

Instructions:

- In a bowl, whisk the honey and lime juice together, until the honey has dissolved.
- Place the slices of watermelon on a large dish.
- Drizzle with the honey-lime dressing, equally.
- Serve immediately.

Watermelon & Lemon Sorbet
Ingredients:

- 8 cups cubed (1 inch) watermelon, seeds and rind discarded 2 Tbsps.
- fresh lemon juice

Instructions:

- In a food processor or blender, puree the watermelon cubes.
- Place 4 cups of the puree in a medium size bowl.
- Stir in the lemon juice
- Freeze it in an ice cream maker. (Use according to the instructions of manufacturer)

Blueberry & Blackberry Yogurt Popsicles
Ingredients:

- 1 cup blueberries
- 1 cup blackberries
- 1 cup non-fat or low-fat plain yogurt
- 1 ¼ cup non-fat or low-fat milk

Instructions:

- Blend the blueberries, blackberries, plain yogurt and milk in a blender.
- Take ½ cup of the smoothie and pour into a Popsicle mold or cups.
- Freeze for half an hour.
- Remove from freezer and insert the Popsicle sticks into the half-frozen smoothie and freeze again until hard. (Approx. 1 hour)

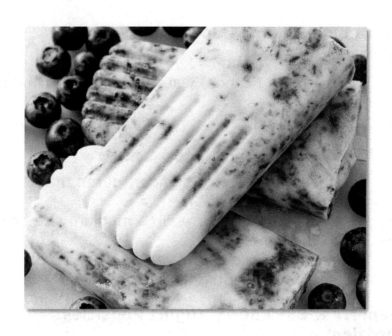

Pumpkin Whip
Ingredients:

- 1 (3.4-oz) package instant sugar-free, fat-free cheesecake-flavor pudding
- 1 cup fat-free milk
- ½ 15-oz can solid pumpkin (not pumpkin pie filling)
- 1 tsp ground cinnamon
- ¼ tsp ground nutmeg ½ 8-oz container sugar-free whipped topping

Instructions:

- In a medium bowl, combine the milk and pudding mix.
- Whisk until it has blended well.
- Add the cinnamon, pumpkin and nutmeg, and stir.
- Mix in the whipped topping, thoroughly.
- Can be served immediately, if not, use plastic wrap to cover and refrigerate. (Can be stored in refrigerator for up to 2 days)

Baked Blueberry Bling
Ingredients:

- 3 cups fresh or frozen blueberries
- 2 tsps. soft salted butter or margarine
- 1 Tbsp. all-purpose flour
- 1 Tbsp. brown sugar
- ½ cup rolled oats
- ½ Tsp. Cinnamon

Instructions:

- Preheat oven at 375°F.
- Wash the blueberries and drain well.
- Arrange the blueberries on a 9-inch pie plate.
- Use a fork to mix the flour, butter, oats, sugar and cinnamon in a small bowl.
- Sprinkle the mixture over the blueberries and bake for 20 to 25 minutes.
- Serve and enjoy while hot.

Pina Colada Popsicles
Ingredients:

- 1 1/3 cups canned diced pineapple, in juice 1/4 cup pineapple juice (from the
- can of pineapple) 1/4 cup sugar
- 1/2 cup light coconut milk
- 1 tsp coconut extract
- 1 Tbsp dark rum (optional)

Instructions:

- Cut the diced pineapple further into chunks.
- Add the pineapple, light coconut milk, sugar, coconut extract and rum, and puree until it is smooth.

- Pour the mixture into Popsicle molds and freeze for about an hour.

Californian Strawberry Dips
Ingredients:

- 4 ½ cups fresh strawberries STRAWBERRY CREAM DIP
- 1/2 cup reduced-fat sour cream
- 1/4 cup strawberries (no sugar added)
- Fruit spread or strawberry jam CHOCOLATE FUDGE DIP
- 6 Tbsps. nonfat yogurt
- 6 Tbsps. prepared chocolate fudge sauce
- 1 1/2 tsps. frozen orange juice concentrate, thawed HONEY ALMOND DIP
- 2/3 cup nonfat yogurt
- 3 Tbsps. toasted, slivered almonds, finely chopped
- 2 1/2 Tbsps. honey

Instructions:

- Wash the strawberries well, drain and pat dry.
- Divide the strawberries equally among 6 dishes and set aside.
- For the dip; whisk the remaining ingredients together until smooth.
- Separate the dip equally among 6 small bowls to accompany each strawberry dish.

Waffle S'mores
Ingredients:

- 8 frozen waffles
- 1 cup Marshmallow Fluff or other marshmallow cream 2–3 Tbsp hot water
- 1/2 cup Nutella or another chocolate-hazelnut spread 1/2 cup semisweet
- chocolate chips 1/2 cup miniature marshmallows

Instructions:

- Toast the waffles until they are crisp.
- Stir the marshmallow fluff with hot water, using a tsp., to make a thick sauce.
- Spread one waffle generously with Nutella, cover with a second waffle, spread more Nutella on top. Repeat with the remaining waffles.
- Drizzle each serving with the marshmallow sauce.
- Top with the chocolate chips and remaining marshmallows.
- Microwave until chips and marshmallows soften. (Approx. 18 to 20 seconds)

Berry-Banana Guilt-Free Ice Cream
Ingredients:

- 3 large bananas, cut into 1-inch pieces and frozen
- 1 cup frozen berries
- 1/2 cup non-fat milk
- 1 1/2 tsps. vanilla extract

Instructions:

- Peel the bananas and slice them.
- Refrigerate overnight or at least 9 hours.
- Remove frozen bananas from the freezer.
- Add the frozen bananas, vanilla and milk in a food processor and process for 2 minutes.
- Stop, and continue to process until it reaches a soft-serve ice cream consistency.
- Add the berries to the processor and blend until pieces of the berries are incorporated into banana mix.
- Serve immediately.

Blueberry & Raspberry Jell-O Parfaits
Ingredients:

- 1 box (3 oz.) raspberry Jell-O
- 1 cup fresh raspberries, plus 4 extras for garnish
  3/4 cup prepared whipped
- topping
- 1 cup fresh blueberries

Instructions:

- In a medium size bowl, stir the Jell-O in with a cup of boiling water.
- Stir for 3 minutes until the Jell-O-O has completely dissolved.
- Stir in a cup of ice water.
- Stir in the raspberries gently.
- Take 4 wine glasses, and divide the mix among them equally using a soup ladle.
- Leave in refrigerator to set for at least 4 hours.
- Take the hardened Jell-O's out of the refrigerator and spread 2 Tbsps. of whipped cream over each of them.
- Garnish each serving with a ¼ cup of blueberries.

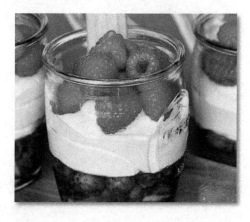

Honey with Lemon Roasted Apples
Ingredients:

- 4 apples
- 2 tbsps. lemon juice
- 1 tbsp. honey
- 1 tbsp. butter, Without salt

Instructions:

- Core apples and cut slices through skin to resemble orange sections. Combine together the honey, lemon juice, and butter.
- Cut up mixture and Serve into apple cores. Wrap apples in lubricated heavy duty aluminum foil, fold up, and seal. Roast until ripe, about 20 minutes. Cut in half to serve.

Special Holiday Spiced Fruit
Ingredients:

- 4 cinnamon sticks
- 20 ounces peaches, drained with juice
- 20 ounces pears, drained with juice
- Half mug Lactose alternative,
- One-Fourth mug cider lemon juice
- 1 tbsp. whole cloves
- 20 ounces pineapple slices, drained with juice

Instructions:

- Merge Lactose alternative, lemon juice, cloves, cinnamon sticks, and fruit juices in big dip saucepan; bring to boil and boil 5 minutes.
- Take off stove and add fruit to syrup. Cool to. Freeze in covered canister at least overnight before using. It keeps for 2 weeks.

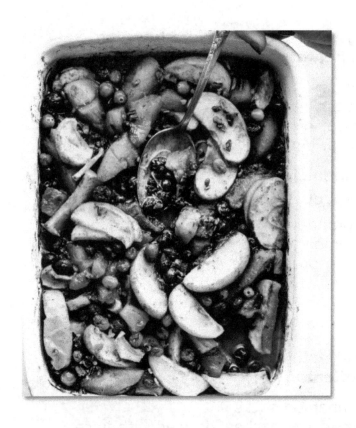

Fresh Fruit Bowl
Ingredients:

- 2 mugs banana, diced
- 2 mugs strawberries,
- 2 peaches, diced
- 1 mug blueberries
- One-Fourth mug Lactose alternative,
- 1 mug low fat vanilla curd

Instructions:

- Merge fruit with Lactose alternative in a big dish. Roll and Shift to a serving dish. Serve with curd.

Frohen Fruit Mus
Ingrediens:

- 12 ounces orange juice concentrate, undiluted
- 2 tbsps. lemon juice
- 17 ounces (485 g) apricot, drained
- 1 mug mineral water
- 1 mug Lactose alternative,
- 30 ounces (840 g) frozen strawberries
- 20 ounces crushed pineapple, drained
- 3 mugs bananas, diced

Instructions:

- Warm up mineral water and Lactose alternative. Add strawberries (juice and all). Add orange juice concentrate and lemon juice. Cut up apricots and add with pineapple and bananas. Put paper muffin holders in muffin tin.
- Cut up mixture among mugs. Put in freezer. After frozen, Take away from pan and store in plastic bags in freezer.

Low Calorie Banana Cake
Ingredients:

- 1 Half mugs (37 g) Lactose alternative,
- 2 eggs
- 1 tsp. vanilla extract
- 1 tsp. lemon juice
- Half mug fat free milk
- Third-Fourth mug (165 g) Without salt butter
- 1 mug mashed bananas
- 2 mugs whole warm up pastry flour
- 1 tsp. baking powder
- Powdered Lactose for dusting

Instructions:

- Combine lemon juice into milk and let stand 5 minutes to sour. Cream butter and Lactose together. Add eggs, milk mixture, vanilla, and bananas.
- Combine until smooth. Whisk together flour and baking powder. Add to creamed combine and combine well.
- Spill into a lubricated baking pan. Bake at 350°F until done, about 35 to 40 minutes. Sprinkle with powdered Lactose if F until you want.

Warm Spiced Fruit Dessert
Ingredients:

- Half mug prunes, stewed
- One-Fourth mug orange marmalade
- One-Fourth tsp. cinnamon
- Half-pound peaches
- Half-pound pears
- Half-pound pineapple
- One-Fourth tsp. nutmeg
- One-Fourth tsp. ground cloves

Instructions:

- Drain liquid from all fruit, reserving Third-Fourth mug (175 g) to make syrup. Merge marmalade, spices, and liquid. Bring to boil and then simmer 3 to 4 minutes.
- Gently add fruit that has been cut into chunks. Shift to slow Oven and Prepare on low at least 4 hours.

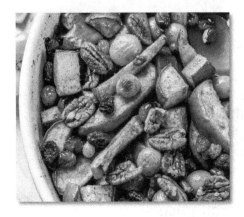

Nicely Spiced Roasted Fruit with ginger
Ingredients:

- 3 tbsps. brown Lactose alternative,
- 1 tsp. cinnamon, ground
- 1 apple
- 1 pear
- 1 banana
- 2 tbsps. Without salt butter, Defrosted
- Half tsp. ground ginger

Instructions:

- Cut the fruit in half or pieces. Do not Peel off. The banana should be cut longitudinally, then in half. Take away the cores.
- Merge butter, brown Lactose alternative, and spices. Baste fruit with mixture. Put fruit on Roast with skin up. Roast on medium-sized 8 to 10 minutes for halves, 4 to 5 minutes for smaller pieces.

Colorful Fruit Mug with Honey
Ingredients:

- 2 bananas, diced
- 10 maraschino cherries, quartered
- 1 apple, cut into small pieces
- 20 ounces pineapple chunks, in juice
- 2 pink grapefruits, sectioned
- 3 oranges, sectioned
- 3 tbsps. Lemon juice
- 2 tsps. Lactose alternative,

Instructions:

- Put pineapple chunks, sectioned grapefruit, and sectioned oranges into big canister. Slice the 2 bananas.
- Cut the apple and cherries. Combine together lemon juice and Splenda. Combine into fruit.

Vanilla Fruit Salad with Honey
Ingredients:

- 1 mug strawberries, halved
- Third-Fourth mug seedless green grapes, halved
- 1 mug blueberries, fresh or frozen softened
- 14 ounces pineapple chunks, in juice
- 11 ounces (310 g) mandarin oranges, undrained
- 1 mug bananas, diced
- 3 Half ounce instant Lactose-free vanilla pudding combine
- Half mug rolled oats, dry fruits, honey

Instructions:

- Drain chunk pineapple and orange segments, reserving liquid in small dish. In big dish, Merge fruits. Sprinkle pudding combine into liquid; combine until Merged and slightly thickened.
- Fold into fruit until well Merged. Serve into serving dishes. Decorate with rolled oats, dry fruits, honey.

CPSIA information can be obtained
at www.ICGtesting.com
Printed in the USA
LVHW080459120521
687183LV00005B/431